EVERYTHING ABOUT LEUKEMIA DIET AND LIFESTYLE CHOICE

Comprehensive Guide To Cancers Of The Blood, Nutrition, Expert Tips For Healthy Living, And Boosting Immunity,

WALTON USELTON

© 2024 [WALTON USELTON]

All rights reserved. No part of this book may be reproduced, distributed, or transmitted in any form or by any means, including photocopying, recording, or other electronic or mechanical methods, without the publisher's prior written permission, with the exception of brief quotations in critical reviews and certain other noncommercial uses permitted by copyright law.

DISCLAIMER

The content in this book is based on the author's expertise and understanding of food and nutrition. The author is not linked or associated with any corporation, business, or person. This book is designed for informative purposes only and should not be interpreted as professional medical advice. Readers should get medical advice before making any changes to their diet or lifestyle. The author takes no responsibility or liability for any repercussions arising from the use of the information included in this book.

Table of Contents

INTRODUCTION 15
- Understanding Leukemia: A Brief Overview......15
- Importance Of Diet And Lifestyle Decisions.......15
- How Can This Book Help You?................................16
- Getting Started: Key Principles.............................17
  - 1. Understanding Nutritional Needs:.................17
  - 2. Hydration:...17
  - 3. Managing Side Effects:....................................18
  - 5. Seeking Professional Guidance:.....................18
- Tips For Success..19
  - 1. Plan Ahead:..19
  - 2. Listen to Your Body:.......................................19
  - 3. Stay Active:..20
  - 4. Self-Care:..20
  - 5. Create a Support Network:............................20

CHAPTER ONE...21
- Understanding Leukemia......................................21
- What Is Leukemia?..21
- Types Of Leukemia...21
- Causes And Risk Factors..22

Symptoms And Diagnoses 23

Treatment Options 24

CHAPTER TWO 27

The Significance Of Diet And Lifestyle Choices . 27

Effects Of Diet On Leukemia 27

The Role Of Exercise In Managing Leukemia 29

Stress Management Techniques 31

Importance Of Sleep 33

Avoiding Harmful Substances 35

CHAPTER THREE 37

Designing A Leukemia Diet 37

The Power Of Plant-Based Foods 37

Incorporating Lean Proteins 38

Choosing Healthy Fats 39

Importance Of Hydration 40

Limit Sugar And Processed Foods 41

CHAPTER FOUR 43

Meal Planning For Leukemia Patients 43

Creating Balanced Meals 43

1. Lean Proteins: 43

2. Whole Grains: 43

3. Fruits and Vegetables: 44
Tips For Cooking Nutritious Foods 45
1. Steaming and sautéing: 45
2. Avoid Overcooking: 46
4. Incorporate Herbs and Spices: 46
5. Limit Processed Foods: 46
Importance Of Portion Control 47
1. Use Smaller Plates: 47
2. Mindful Eating: 47
3. Measure Portions: 48
4. Avoid Seconds: 48
5. Balance the Plate: 48
Snack Ideas For Energy Boost 49
1. Greek Yoghurt with Berries: 49
2. Nut Butter with Apple Slices: 49
3. Hummus with Veggie Sticks: 49
5. Smoothies: 50
Meal Preparation Strategies For Busy Days 50
1. Prepare Ahead: 50
4. Use Freezer-Friendly Recipes: 51
5. Preparing Ingredients: 52

6. Use Slow Cookers and Instant Pots: 52

CHAPTER FIVE 53

Nutrients That Support Leukemia Treatment .. 53

Antioxidants: Their Role 53

    Sources of antioxidants: 53

    How To Incorporate Antioxidants: 54

Essential Vitamins And Minerals 54

    Key vitamins: 55

    Important Minerals: 55

    Practical tips: 56

Omega-3 Fatty Acid Benefits 56

    Sources of omega-3 fatty acids: 57

    How To Incorporate Omega-3s: 57

Fibre Promotes Digestive Health 58

    Types of Fibre: 58

    Benefits of Fibre: 59

    Practical Methods to Increase Fibre Intake: .. 59

Adaptogenic Herbs And Supplements 60

    Popular adaptogenic herbs: 60

    Supplements to consider: 61

    How to use adaptogens: 61

CHAPTER SIX 63
Exercise And Physical Activity 63
Benefits Of Exercise For Patients With Leukemia
.... 63
Types Of Exercises To Consider 64
Incorporating Movement Into Daily Routines .. 66
Overcoming Barriers To Exercise 67
Working With A Healthcare Team To Ensure Safe Exercise 68

CHAPTER SEVEN 69
Stress-Management Techniques........................... 69
Mindfulness Meditation.. 69
Deep Breathing Exercises 70
Yoga And Tai Chi For Relaxation 71
Stress Relief Through Creative Activities 72
Seeking Support From Loved Ones 73

CHAPTER EIGHT 75
The Importance Of Quality Sleep.......................... 75
Understanding Sleep Patterns 75
Creating A Restful Sleep Environment 76
Sleep Hygiene Practices... 77

- Managing Sleep Disturbances 78
- Seeking Professional Help With Sleep Issues 79

CHAPTER NINE 81
- Avoiding Harmful Substances 81
- Effects Of Smoking And Alcohol 81
- Risks Of Environmental Toxins 82
- Importance Of Medication Compliance 84
- Herbal Supplements To Avoid 85
- Creating A Healthy Environment At Home 86

CHAPTER TEN 89
- Ensuring Long-Term Health And Wellness 89
- Regular Monitoring And Follow-Up 89
- Changing Diet And Lifestyle Over Time 91
- Finding Joy In Everyday Life 92
- Celebrating Progress And Achievements 94
- Continuing Education And Support Network 96
- CONCLUSION 99

THE END 101

ABOUT THIS BOOK

"Leukemia Diet And Lifestyle Choice" is a thorough book that provides essential insights into the critical interaction between diet, lifestyle, and leukemia treatment. As the title indicates, this book dives into the complex relationship between what we eat, how we live, and how these factors influence leukemia outcomes. This book, which explores all aspects of leukemia management, from comprehending the illness to practical recommendations for implementing healthy behaviors, acts as a beacon of empowerment for patients, carers, and healthcare professionals alike.

This book begins with a clear and straightforward introduction to leukemia, explaining its many forms, causes, symptoms, diagnosis, and treatment choices. This core knowledge prepares readers to comprehend the need to take a proactive approach to illness management.

This book's theme is the importance of food and lifestyle choices in minimizing the effects of leukemia. Chapter 2 digs further into this subject, revealing the tremendous impact of food, exercise, stress management, sleep, and avoiding dangerous drugs on leukemia results. By emphasizing the significance of overall well-being, this book encourages readers to take control of their health.

One noteworthy element of "Leukemia Diet And Lifestyle Choice" is its practical approach to making nutritional adjustments. Chapter 3 walks readers through the process of creating a leukemia-friendly diet, promoting the inclusion of plant-based meals, lean proteins, healthy fats, enough water, and limiting sugar and processed foods. Furthermore, Chapter 4 provides crucial meal planning tools and nutritional dishes customized to the requirements of leukemia patients, ensuring that they are well nourished.

Recognizing the importance of certain foods in leukemia therapy, Chapter 5 investigates the advantages of antioxidants, critical vitamins and minerals, omega-3 fatty acids, fiber, and adaptogenic herbs. This evidence-based approach teaches readers how to make educated food choices that support their medical therapy.

In addition to nutritional concerns, this book emphasizes the necessity of regular exercise, stress management skills, enough sleep, and avoiding dangerous drugs to boost general well-being. Chapters 6-9 provide practical recommendations and concrete guidance for incorporating these lifestyle changes into everyday life, boosting resilience and promoting optimum health outcomes.

Finally, "Leukemia Diet And Lifestyle Choice" extends beyond illness treatment to emphasize the value of long-term health and well-being. Chapter 10 urges readers to adopt a continuous-improvement mentality, recognize accomplishments, and build a supporting network for continued encouragement and direction.

In essence, "Leukemia Diet And Lifestyle Choice" goes beyond the scope of a standard health guide, providing a comprehensive road map for empowerment, resilience, and well-being in the face of leukemia. This book provides readers with information, resources, and inspiration, acting as a beacon of hope and empowerment on the path to maximum health and vitality.

INTRODUCTION

Understanding Leukemia: A Brief Overview

Leukemia is a malignancy that affects the blood and bone marrow, which create blood cells. It is characterized by the overproduction of aberrant white blood cells, which push out good cells and weaken the body's capacity to fight infection. There are several forms of leukemia, each with unique features and treatment techniques. Some frequent kinds include acute myeloid leukemia (AML), acute lymphoblastic leukemia (ALL), chronic myeloid leukemia (CML), and chronic lymphocytic leukemia (CLL).

Importance Of Diet And Lifestyle Decisions

While medical therapies like chemotherapy, radiation therapy, and bone marrow transplants are critical in the treatment of leukemia, nutrition, and lifestyle choices also play an important role in maintaining general health and well-being throughout treatment. A well-balanced, nutrient-dense diet may help strengthen the immune system, maintain energy levels, control treatment adverse effects, and encourage overall recovery. Similarly, adopting good lifestyle habits like regular exercise, stress management, and getting enough sleep may boost the body's resilience and improve quality of life.

How Can This Book Help You?

This book seeks to offer practical advice and information for those impacted by leukemia, whether they are patients, carers, or family members. By investigating the link between nutrition, lifestyle, and leukemia management, readers will obtain useful insights into making educated decisions that may improve their health and treatment results. This book provides a complete approach to holistic well-being in the context of leukemia care, including nutritional suggestions, meal planning ideas, exercise regimens, and stress-relief tactics.

Getting Started: Key Principles

1. **Understanding Nutritional Needs:** Proper nutrition is critical for the body's capacity to deal with leukemia and its treatment. This involves eating a range of nutrient-dense meals to fulfill energy needs, maintain muscle mass, and boost immunological function. Include lean proteins, whole grains, fruits, vegetables, and healthy fats in your meals to guarantee a well-rounded diet.

2. **Hydration:** Staying hydrated is critical for those receiving leukemia treatment because it helps flush out toxins, regulates body temperature, and prevents dehydration. Drink lots of fluids throughout the day, including water, herbal teas, and electrolyte-rich

beverages, but avoid excessive coffee and sugary drinks.

3. Managing Side Effects: Treatments for leukemia, such as chemotherapy and radiation therapy, may induce nausea, appetite changes, mouth sores, and exhaustion. To reduce these symptoms, consider changing your diet to include smaller, more often meals, eating bland or easily digested foods, and using anti-nausea medicines advised by your healthcare team.

4. Mindful Eating entails paying attention to your body's hunger and fullness signals, as well as enjoying the flavors and sensations of your meal. This strategy may improve digestion, decrease overeating, and increase overall meal satisfaction, especially during difficult circumstances.

5. Seeking Professional Guidance: While broad dietary suggestions might be beneficial, it is critical to speak with a licensed dietitian or nutritionist who specializes in cancer treatment for personalized guidance suited to your unique requirements and desires. They can provide professional advice on managing nutritional shortages, dietary restrictions, and food-related issues during your leukemia treatment.

Tips For Success

1. **Plan Ahead:** Take the time to plan your meals and snacks, taking into account your treatment schedule, dietary preferences, and nutritional objectives. Stock up on pantry basics, fresh vegetables, and nutritious convenience items to make meal preparation simpler on hectic days or when you're not feeling well.

2. **Listen to Your Body:** Consider how various meals make you feel and change your diet appropriately. If specific meals cause digestive pain or aggravate side effects, choose better-tolerated alternatives or see a healthcare practitioner.

3. Stay Active: Incorporating regular physical exercise into your routine will help you gain energy, improve your mood, and feel better overall. Choose activities that are enjoyable and appropriate for your fitness level, such as walking, swimming, yoga, or lightweight training.

4. Self-Care: Managing leukemia may be physically and emotionally demanding, therefore it's important to prioritize self-care activities that encourage relaxation and stress reduction. Find what works best for you, whether it's meditation, deep breathing exercises, outdoor activities, or hobbies, and make time for it regularly.

5. Create a Support Network: Surround yourself with supportive friends, family members, and healthcare professionals who understand your situation and can provide encouragement, direction, and practical aid as required.

CHAPTER ONE

Understanding Leukemia

What Is Leukemia?

Leukemia is a malignancy that affects both the blood and bone marrow. Normally, the bone marrow produces white blood cells, which are essential for fighting infections; red blood cells, which transport oxygen throughout the body; and platelets, which aid in blood clotting. However, in leukemia, the bone marrow generates aberrant white blood cells that do not function correctly and increase rapidly. These aberrant cells may crowd out regular blood cells, causing a range of health issues.

Types Of Leukemia

There are various forms of leukemia, however, they are divided into four categories: acute There are four types of leukemia: acute myeloid leukemia (AML), chronic myeloid leukemia (CLL), and lymphocytic leukemia (ALL). Each form of leukemia affects various types of white blood cells and has distinct features and treatment options.

Acute leukemia advances quickly and needs prompt treatment, but chronic leukemia progresses slowly and may not require treatment right immediately. Furthermore, leukemia may be categorized depending on the precise kind of white blood cell involved, among other characteristics.

Causes And Risk Factors

The actual etiology of leukemia is unknown, however, some risk factors enhance the probability of having the condition. These risk factors include exposure to certain chemicals (such as benzene), radiation exposure, genetic factors (such as a family history of leukemia), medical problems (such as Down syndrome), and certain forms of chemotherapy or radiation treatment used to treat other malignancies.

It is crucial to emphasize that not everyone with these risk factors will acquire leukemia, and some leukemia patients may have no recognized risk factors.

Symptoms And Diagnoses

The symptoms of leukemia vary depending on the kind of leukemia and other variables. Common symptoms include tiredness, weakness, recurrent infections, fever, easy bruising or bleeding, enlarged lymph nodes, and unexplained weight loss. However, some leukemia patients may not exhibit any symptoms in the early stages of the illness.

Leukemia is normally diagnosed using a combination of medical history, physical examination, blood testing, and bone marrow assays. These tests may assist assess the kind and severity of leukemia, which is essential for designing an effective treatment strategy.

Treatment Options

Treatment for leukemia is determined by various criteria, including the kind of leukemia, the patient's age and general health, and the severity of the illness. Common treatment methods include chemotherapy, targeted therapy, radiation therapy, immunotherapy, and stem cell transplantation.

The objective of therapy is to kill leukemia cells while restoring normal blood cell production. In certain situations, therapy may result in full remission, which means there is no sign of leukemia in the body. However, certain kinds of leukemia are more difficult to cure or may recur after a time of remission.

Patients with leukemia should collaborate closely with their healthcare team to build a personalized treatment plan that takes into account their unique requirements and preferences. Furthermore, continuing monitoring and follow-up care are often required to track the condition and manage any possible adverse effects of therapy.

CHAPTER TWO

The Significance Of Diet And Lifestyle Choices

Effects Of Diet On Leukemia

When it comes to leukemia, nutrition is critical in maintaining general health and treating the disease. A well-balanced diet may help strengthen the immune system, boost energy levels, and improve general health. But what should this diet consist of?

First, be sure to include enough fruits and veggies in your meals. These colorful foods are high in critical vitamins, minerals, and antioxidants, which may help improve immunity and fight illnesses. Aim for a diversity of colors to ensure you obtain a diverse assortment of nutrients.

Next, include lean protein sources in your diet, such as chicken, fish, beans, and tofu. Protein is required for tissue growth and repair, which is particularly critical for those receiving leukemia therapies.

Whole grains should also be a mainstay in your diet. Choose whole grain bread, pasta, rice, and oats, which are high in fiber and include essential elements like iron and B vitamins. Fibre helps aid digestion and reduce constipation, which is a typical side effect of leukemia therapy.

Remember to include healthy fats in your diet, such as avocados, nuts, seeds, and olive oil. These fats are essential for brain function, hormone synthesis, and inflammation reduction in the body.

Finally, remain hydrated by drinking lots of water all day. Proper hydration is necessary for general health and may aid in the removal of toxins from the body.

A balanced diet rich in fruits, vegetables, lean proteins, whole grains, and healthy fats may help your body's natural defenses and enhance your overall quality of life while living with leukemia.

The Role Of Exercise In Managing Leukemia

Exercise is another vital part of controlling leukemia and improving general health. Regular physical exercise may boost strength, endurance, and happiness while decreasing weariness and stress.

For patients receiving leukemia therapy, it is critical to begin carefully and progressively increase the intensity and duration of exercise as tolerated. Even mild activities such as walking, yoga, and swimming may be quite beneficial.

Strength training activities, such as lifting weights or using resistance bands, may assist in retaining muscle mass and bone density, which may be lost after therapy.

Cardiovascular workouts, such as bicycling or running, may benefit heart health and circulation while also increasing energy and lowering weariness.

Exercise may also improve mental health by lowering anxiety, sadness, and stress. It may create a feeling of success and empowerment, which is particularly crucial when dealing with a difficult diagnosis such as leukemia.

Remember to listen to your body and talk with your doctor before beginning any new workout regimen. They may advise you on safe and suitable activities depending on your specific health state and treatment plan.

Regular exercise may make you feel stronger, more energized, and better prepared to face the difficulties of life with leukemia.

Stress Management Techniques

Stress management is critical for general health, particularly for leukemia patients. High amounts of stress may impair the immune system, worsen symptoms, and disrupt treatment results. Fortunately, there are several effective methods for lowering stress and increasing relaxation.

Deep breathing exercises are one of the easiest strategies to reduce stress. Practice taking slow, deep breaths, concentrating on filling your lungs with air before gently expelling. This may assist in stimulating the body's relaxation response and quiet the mind.

Mindfulness meditation is another effective stress-management technique. This entails paying attention to the current moment without judgment and letting ideas and sensations pass without becoming engrossed in them. Regular meditation has been demonstrated to alleviate stress, anxiety, and depression while enhancing general mental health.

Participating in things you like may also assist to reduce stress and improve mood. Whether it's reading, gardening, painting, or performing music, making time for hobbies and interests may give a much-needed reprieve from the stresses of daily life.

Physical exercise is another great approach to relieving stress. Endorphins, which work as natural pain relievers and mood lifters in the brain, are released during exercise. Even a brief stroll or light yoga practice might help to raise your mood and decrease stress.

Finally, never underestimate the value of social support. Spending time with loved ones, chatting with friends, or joining a support group may all give emotional and practical help during tough times.

Incorporating these stress management tactics into your daily routine can help you deal with the difficulties of living with leukemia and enhance your overall quality of life.

Importance Of Sleep

Getting adequate sleep is critical for general health and well-being, particularly for those with leukemia. Quality sleep improves immune function, emotional control, and energy levels, making it critical for symptom management and recovery.

Setting a consistent sleep pattern may assist regulate your body's internal clock and enhance the quality of your sleep. Aim to go to bed and wake up at the same time every day, including weekends, to help teach your body to fall asleep and wake up more easily.

Creating a peaceful bedtime ritual might also signal to your body that it's time to unwind and get ready for sleep. This might involve taking a warm bath, reading a book, or practicing relaxation methods such as deep breathing or meditation.

It's also critical to design a sleep-friendly atmosphere in your bedroom. Keep the room cold, dark, and quiet, and invest in a good mattress and pillows for maximum comfort and support.

Limiting screen time before bedtime is another critical component of establishing excellent sleep hygiene. Phones, tablets, and laptops produce blue light, which may affect the synthesis of melatonin, a hormone that governs sleep-wake cycles. Try to avoid devices for at least an hour before sleep to allow your brain to relax.

If you're having trouble sleeping because of leukemia symptoms or side effects, speak with your doctor. They may provide advice on how to manage sleep disruptions and may prescribe techniques or drugs to assist improve sleep quality.

Prioritizing sleep and developing good sleep habits will help your body's natural healing processes and enhance your overall quality of life while living with leukemia.

Avoiding Harmful Substances

When living with leukemia, it's critical to avoid dangerous chemicals that might worsen symptoms and interfere with therapy. This includes tobacco smoke, which contains a variety of carcinogens that may raise the chance of getting leukemia and other cancers.

If you smoke, quitting is one of the most beneficial things you can do for your health. Quitting is never too late, and it may dramatically lower your chance of acquiring leukemia problems while also improving your general quality of life.

Secondhand smoke is equally dangerous and should be avoided whenever feasible. If you are exposed to smoke at your home or office, make efforts to reduce your exposure or seek out smoke-free settings to spend time in.

Alcohol use should also be minimized or avoided since it might impair the body's capacity to metabolize drugs and worsen some adverse effects of leukemia therapy. If you choose to consume alcohol, do it in moderation and always listen to your healthcare team's advice.

Other substances to avoid include recreational drugs and some medicines that may interfere with leukemia treatments. Always contact your healthcare provider before starting any new drugs or supplements to verify they are safe and suitable for your specific needs.

Avoiding dangerous drugs and adopting a healthy lifestyle will help your body's natural healing processes and enhance your overall quality of life while living with leukemia.

CHAPTER THREE

Designing A Leukemia Diet

The Power Of Plant-Based Foods

When it comes to constructing a healthy diet, plant-based foods are your greatest friend. Fruits, vegetables, whole grains, legumes, nuts, and seeds are high in critical vitamins, minerals, antioxidants, and phytochemicals, which may help strengthen your immune system and attack leukemia cells. These meals include a variety of nutrients that your body needs to remain healthy and powerful throughout treatment.

One of the primary advantages of plant-based diets is their high fiber content. Fiber aids digestion, supports healthy bowel motions, and may even reduce cholesterol levels.

Furthermore, many plant-based meals are low in calories and saturated fat, making them perfect for maintaining a healthy weight.

Adding more plant-based items to your diet is simpler than you may think. Begin by filling half of your plate with fruits and veggies for each meal. Choose a variety of colors to ensure you obtain a diverse spectrum of nutrients. Snack on fresh fruits, raw veggies, or nuts throughout the day to stay energized and satisfied.

Incorporating Lean Proteins

While plant-based foods should be the cornerstone of your leukemia diet, it is also critical to include lean proteins to promote muscle building and repair. Lean proteins such as chicken, turkey, fish, tofu, and lentils are high in necessary amino acids, which are the building blocks of protein.

When it comes to protein sources, consider lean cuts of meat and poultry, as well as omega-3-rich seafood like salmon and trout. Tofu, tempeh, lentils, chickpeas, and black beans are all excellent plant-based protein alternatives. These meals not only include protein but also other essential elements such as iron and zinc.

To integrate lean proteins into your meals, consider adding grilled chicken breast to salads, using beans or lentils in soups and stews, or eating baked fish with steamed veggies. Experiment with various recipes and cooking techniques to keep your meals interesting and delectable.

Choosing Healthy Fats

While fats have a negative reputation, not all fats are created equal. In reality, healthy fats are an important component of a well-balanced diet, particularly for those with leukemia. Healthy fats give concentrated energy, promote cell development and repair, and aid in the absorption of fat-soluble vitamins A, D, E, and K.

When selecting fats for your leukemia diet, look for sources of unsaturated fats such as olive oil, avocado, almonds, and seeds. These fats have been demonstrated to decrease inflammation, cut cholesterol, and improve cardiovascular health. Avoid trans fats and restrict saturated fats, which may raise the risk of heart disease and other health issues.

To add healthy fats to your diet, use olive oil as a salad dressing or a cooking oil while sautéing veggies. For a healthy breakfast or snack, try a handful of almonds or walnuts, or spread avocado over whole-grain bread. By selecting healthy fats, you may improve the flavor of your meals while also benefiting your general health.

Importance Of Hydration

Maintaining hydration is critical for everyone, but it is particularly vital for those with leukemia. Proper hydration promotes healthy blood volume, regulates body temperature, and eliminates toxins. Dehydration may increase symptoms such as tiredness, nausea, and constipation, so stay hydrated throughout the day.

Water is the greatest option for remaining hydrated, but you may also drink herbal tea, broth, and diluted fruit juice. Aim to drink at least eight glasses of water every day, and increase your fluid intake if you have symptoms such as vomiting or diarrhea.

In addition to drinking fluids, you may boost your water consumption by eating water-rich meals such as fruits and vegetables. Cucumbers, watermelon, strawberries, and spinach are all good sources of water. Incorporating these items into your meals and snacks will help you stay hydrated and healthy.

Limit Sugar And Processed Foods

While it is vital to include nutritional items in your leukemia diet, it is also critical to restrict or avoid meals heavy in sugar and processed substances.

Excess sugar consumption has been related to inflammation, insulin resistance, and an increased risk of chronic illnesses such as diabetes and heart disease.

Processed foods, such as fast food, frozen meals, and packaged snacks, often include extra sugars, bad fats, and artificial additives that may be detrimental to your health. These meals are low in nutritional content and may lead to weight gain and other health issues.

Instead of sugary snacks or processed meals, choose whole, minimally processed foods wherever feasible. Choose fresh fruits and vegetables, whole grains, lean proteins, and healthy fats to fuel your body and promote overall health. Making attentive food choices may help you optimize your nutrition and assist your body's natural capacity to fight leukemia.

CHAPTER FOUR

Meal Planning For Leukemia Patients

Creating Balanced Meals

When preparing meals for leukemia patients, it's critical to prioritize a balanced diet that promotes general health and helps control treatment adverse effects. A well-balanced meal has a range of dietary categories, such as lean proteins, whole grains, fruits and vegetables, and healthy fats.

1. **Lean Proteins:** Include foods like chicken, turkey, fish, eggs, tofu, beans, and lentils. Proteins are essential for tissue repair and immunological response. For example, grilled chicken breast or bean salad might be excellent protein sources.

2. **Whole Grains:** Opt for whole grains such as brown rice, quinoa, whole wheat pasta, and oats over

processed grains. Whole grains include fiber, which promotes digestion and maintains energy levels. A plate of quinoa salad or a bowl of muesli with berries might be a great way to start.

3. Fruits and Vegetables: Choose a diversity of colors in fruits and vegetables to provide a wide range of vitamins and minerals. Dark leafy greens, berries, carrots, and citrus fruits are especially nutrient-rich. Steamed broccoli or a fresh fruit salad may be both delicious and healthy.

4. Avocados, almonds, seeds, and olive oil are all good sources of healthy fats. Healthy fats are necessary for brain function and may help reduce inflammation. A tiny handful of nuts or a sprinkle of olive oil over a salad might boost the meal's nutritious value.

Consider designing a meal like a plate with separate parts for each food type. For example, a dinner plate may include grilled salmon (protein), brown rice (whole grain), steamed asparagus, and carrots (vegetables), as well as a small side salad topped with avocado (good fat).

Tips For Cooking Nutritious Foods

Cooking techniques have a considerable influence on the nutritious content of meals. Here are some strategies to ensure you're making meals that keep the most nutrients:

1. **Steaming and sautéing:** These procedures maintain more nutrients than boiling. Steaming veggies, such as broccoli and carrots, preserve their vitamins and minerals. Sautéing with a little olive oil may improve flavor without sacrificing nutritional value.

2. **Avoid Overcooking:** Overcooking may destroy key nutrients, especially in vegetables. Cook them till just tender but still brilliant in color. For example, stir-frying bell peppers for a few minutes keeps them crisp and rich in vitamin C.

3. Whenever possible, utilize fresh, seasonal vegetables. Fresh products often have more nutrients than canned or processed alternatives. For example, fresh tomato sauce produced from ripe tomatoes will be more nutrient-dense than canned tomato sauce.

4. **Incorporate Herbs and Spices:** Herbs and spices not only enhance flavor but also provide health advantages. Turmeric, ginger, garlic, and basil may improve foods while also offering anti-inflammatory and antioxidant benefits. A pinch of turmeric in a lentil soup or fresh basil in a salad may enhance both flavor and nutrition.

5. **Limit Processed Foods:** Processed foods often include extra sugars, harmful fats, and salt. Concentrate on

entire meals that are as near to their original form as possible. Instead of a prepackaged snack, try an apple with peanut butter or a handmade trail mix.

Importance Of Portion Control

Portion management is essential for keeping a healthy weight and ensuring that the body receives the necessary nutrients without overeating. Here are some helpful strategies for controlling portions:

1. **Use Smaller Plates:** Smaller plates might help you regulate portion sizes and avoid overeating. Filling a smaller plate creates the appearance of more food, which helps with contentment.

2. **Mindful Eating:** Pay attention to your hunger signs and eat gently. This helps to prevent overeating since it takes the brain around 20 minutes to detect fullness. Chewing food carefully and savoring each mouthful might help you enjoy your meals and avoid overeating.

3. Measure Portions: Use measuring cups or a food scale to guarantee correct portion proportions, particularly if you're new to portion management. For example, a portion of cooked pasta should be around half a cup, whereas a dish of lean meat should be about the size of a deck of cards.

4. Avoid Seconds: Begin with a single dish and wait before choosing if you want more. When your body signals fullness, the original quantity is usually adequate.

5. Balance the Plate: Aim to fill half of your plate with veggies, one-quarter with protein, and one-quarter with complete grains. This visual guide may help you maintain balanced quantities and avoid overconsumption of any food category.

Snack Ideas For Energy Boost

Snacking may be an important element of maintaining energy levels, particularly for leukemia patients who may feel fatigued. Here are some nutritious, energy-boosting snack ideas:

1. **Greek Yoghurt with Berries:** Greek yogurt contains protein and calcium, while berries provide antioxidants and vitamins. This mixture is both refreshing and nourishing.

2. **Nut Butter with Apple Slices:** Apples include fiber and vitamins, while nut butter has healthy fats and protein. This combination results in a tasty and energizing snack.

3. **Hummus with Veggie Sticks:** Carrots, celery, and bell peppers combined with hummus make for a crunchy and nutritious snack. Hummus is high in protein and healthy fats, making it an excellent source of sustained energy.

4. Trail Mix: A combination of nuts, seeds, and dried fruits may be a quick and calorie-dense snack. Choose unsweetened and unsalted types to keep it healthy. A handful of trail mix may deliver a rapid energy boost without any added sugar or salt.

5. Smoothies: Combine fruits, vegetables, and a protein source, such as Greek yogurt or protein powder, for a fast and healthy snack. Spinach, banana, and almond milk form a delightful and energizing smoothie.

Meal Preparation Strategies For Busy Days

Meal planning may assist leukemia patients in maintaining a nutritious diet even on hectic days. Here are some tips to make meal preparation simpler and more efficient:

1. Prepare Ahead: Take some time each week to prepare meals and snacks. Create a shopping list to ensure you have all of the required materials.

This minimizes the possibility of choosing unhealthy alternatives owing to a shortage of time.

2. Batch cooking involves preparing huge amounts of basic items such as grains, proteins, and vegetables. For example, make a large quantity of quinoa, grill a few chicken breasts, and bake a tray of mixed veggies. These may be kept in the fridge and blended throughout the week.

3. Divide prepared items into single-serving containers. When time is of the essence, you may easily grab a pre-portioned meal or snack. Clear containers allow you to see what is within at a glance.

4. **Use Freezer-Friendly Recipes:** Prepare dishes that store well, such as soups, stews, and casseroles. Place these meals in freezer-safe containers for convenient reheating. For example, a large batch of vegetable lentil soup may be split and stored for later use.

5. Preparing Ingredients: Wash, cut, and store fresh fruits and vegetables ahead of time. This makes it simple to put together meals and snacks fast. For example, having pre-chopped vegetables on hand might make preparing a stir-fry or salad easier.

6. Use Slow Cookers and Instant Pots: These appliances may save you time and effort by enabling you to make meals with little hands-on time. Place the ingredients in a slow cooker in the morning and return home to a ready-to-eat supper.

Leukaemia sufferers may maintain a balanced diet that maintains their health and energy levels while undergoing treatment and going about their everyday lives by following these methods and ideas.

CHAPTER FIVE

Nutrients That Support Leukemia Treatment

Antioxidants: Their Role

Antioxidants are substances that protect cells from free radicals, which are unstable molecules that may damage cellular structures and lead to cancer formation. Incorporating antioxidants into leukemia patients' diets may assist in strengthening their body's defense systems during treatment.

Sources of antioxidants:

• Blueberries, strawberries, spinach, kale, and bell peppers contain antioxidants such as vitamin C and flavonoids.

• Nuts and seeds: Almonds, walnuts, and sunflower seeds contain vitamin E, a potent antioxidant.

- Green tea contains catechins, powerful antioxidants that may boost immunological function.

How To Incorporate Antioxidants:

- Create a nutrient-dense smoothie by blending berries, spinach, and almonds.

- Make colorful salads with spinach, bell peppers, and almonds. Add a citrus-based dressing for an added dose of vitamin C.

- Healthy snack options include nuts and seeds.

By eating antioxidant-rich foods regularly, leukemia patients may help their bodies regulate oxidative stress, perhaps improving treatment results and general health.

Essential Vitamins And Minerals

Certain vitamins and minerals are essential for boosting the immune system, promoting healing, and guaranteeing general well-being throughout leukemia therapy.

Key vitamins:

- Vitamin C boosts immunological function and improves iron absorption. Citrus fruits, strawberries, and broccoli all contain this.

- Vitamin D promotes bone health and immunological response. Fortified dairy products, fatty seafood such as salmon, and sunshine exposure are also potential sources.

- B vitamins promote energy generation and red blood cell development. Whole grains, legumes, and green leafy vegetables are good sources of iron.

Important Minerals:

- Iron is crucial for red blood cell formation, which may be affected during leukemia therapy. Found in lean meats, legumes, and fortified grains.

- Calcium is crucial for bone health, especially for those on steroids. Found in dairy products, plant milks that have been supplemented and leafy greens.

• Magnesium promotes muscular and nerve function, as well as energy metabolism. Found in nuts, seeds, and whole grains.

Practical tips:

• Include a variety of food categories in each meal to ensure adequate vitamin and mineral intake.

• Fortified meals, such as cereals and plant-based milks, may help increase nutritional intake.

• Consult a healthcare professional for recommended vitamin and mineral supplements if food consumption is inadequate.

Omega-3 Fatty Acid Benefits

Omega-3 fatty acids are necessary fats that have been demonstrated to lower inflammation and improve general health, which is especially good for leukemia patients under chemotherapy.

Sources of omega-3 fatty acids:

- Fatty fish, such as salmon, mackerel, and sardines, have high levels of DHA and EPA, which are omega-3s.

Flaxseeds, chia seeds, and walnuts contain ALA, a plant-based omega-3.

- Supplements: Fish oil and algae oil may augment omega-3 consumption if dietary sources are inadequate.

How To Incorporate Omega-3s:

- Incorporate fatty fish into your diet at least twice a week. Baked or grilled fish may be a tasty and nutritious meal.

- Increase omega-3 intake by adding ground flaxseeds or chia seeds to smoothies.

- Walnuts are a versatile snack that may be added to salads or muesli.

Regular omega-3 fatty acid intake may help regulate inflammation, promote cardiovascular health, and perhaps improve the efficacy of leukemia therapies.

Fibre Promotes Digestive Health

Dietary fiber is vital for maintaining a healthy digestive tract, which is especially important for leukemia patients who may develop gastrointestinal disorders as a result of their therapy.

Types of Fibre:

• Soluble fiber is found in oats, beans, and fruits such as apples and berries. It helps to manage blood sugar levels and reduces cholesterol.

• Insoluble fiber is found in whole grains, nuts, and vegetables. It increases the volume of the stool and promotes regular bowel motions.

Benefits of Fibre:

- Regular digestion prevents constipation, a major concern during cancer therapy.

- Blood Sugar Control: Maintaining stable blood sugar levels may improve general health.

- Promotes satiety, aiding in weight management.

Practical Methods to Increase Fibre Intake:

- Choose whole-grain bread, pasta, and cereals over refined alternatives.

- Incorporate a variety of fruits and vegetables in each meal. Aim for a minimum of five servings each day.

- Incorporate legumes like beans, lentils, and chickpeas into soups, salads, and stews.

Leukemia sufferers may improve their gut health and tolerance to therapies by consuming enough fiber.

Adaptogenic Herbs And Supplements

Adaptogenic herbs are natural chemicals that assist the body cope with stress and maintain general equilibrium. They may be especially helpful for leukemia patients struggling with the physical and mental stresses of treatment.

Popular adaptogenic herbs:

• Ashwagandha is known for its stress-reduction and immune-boosting benefits.

• Rhodiola Rosea: Reduces tiredness and enhances physical and mental performance.

• Turmeric (Curcumin) has anti-inflammatory qualities that may help decrease inflammation after cancer therapy.

Supplements to consider:

• Probiotics promote gut health and immunological function. Found in yogurt and available as a supplement.

• Milk Thistle has liver-protective qualities, making it advantageous for chemotherapy patients.

• Reishi Mushroom: Improves immune function and has anti-cancer qualities.

How to use adaptogens:

• Use herbal teas to include adaptogenic herbs into your diet. For example, ashwagandha tea may be both relaxing and helpful.

• Consult a healthcare professional for the proper dose and form of adaptogenic supplements.

• Use turmeric in cooking. It may be used in soups, stews, and smoothies.

Leukemia patients may boost their body's resilience by including adaptogenic herbs and vitamins in their daily routine, possibly enhancing their treatment response and overall quality of life.

CHAPTER SIX

Exercise And Physical Activity

Benefits Of Exercise For Patients With Leukemia

Exercise is an essential component of leukemia treatment, providing several advantages that help general well-being. Regular physical exercise may increase energy, reduce tiredness, and enhance mood, all of which are significant issues for leukemia patients. Exercise also strengthens the immune system, improving the body's capacity to fight infections, which is especially essential for those who have impaired immune systems as a result of leukemia or its treatment.

Furthermore, exercise is essential for preserving cardiovascular function, which might be compromised by some leukemia therapies.

It increases heart and lung function, improves circulation, and lowers the risk of cardiovascular illness. Exercise also helps to maintain a healthy body weight and muscle mass, which counteracts the muscle withering and weight loss that many leukemia patients endure.

Furthermore, physical exercise may help with stress and anxiety, providing a constructive outlet for mental well-being. It may help people deal with the psychological obstacles of leukemia diagnosis and treatment by instilling a feeling of empowerment and control over their health.

Types Of Exercises To Consider

Leukemia patients should do a range of activities that include aerobic, strength, flexibility, and balance training. Aerobic workouts including walking, running, cycling, and swimming improve cardiovascular fitness and endurance.

They also increase oxygen circulation throughout the body, which improves energy levels and general health.

Strength training activities, such as weightlifting or utilizing resistance bands, aid in the development and maintenance of muscular mass. This is especially essential in treating muscular weakness and exhaustion, which are often linked with leukemia and its therapies. Flexibility activities, like yoga or stretching regimens, improve joint mobility and avoid stiffness, resulting in greater movement and functioning.

Balance activities, such as tai chi or particular yoga positions, enhance stability and coordination, lowering the chance of falling. This is especially important for leukemia patients, who may feel dizziness or weakness as a result of treatment side effects.

Incorporating Movement Into Daily Routines

To receive the advantages of exercise constantly, leukemia patients must include physical activity in their daily routines. Simple tactics like going for short walks, using the stairs instead of the lift, and gardening may build up to large amounts of movement over time. Setting attainable objectives, such as aiming for a particular number of steps per day or allotting a set amount of time for exercise, may help develop a habit and keep motivation.

To guarantee long-term commitment, activities must be both pleasurable and sustainable. Experimenting with various types of exercise and determining what feels best for individual tastes and physical abilities is essential. Incorporating movement into regular tasks, such as doing housework or playing with dogs, may help exercise seem more natural and simple.

Overcoming Barriers To Exercise

Leukemia patients may confront a variety of challenges to exercise, including weariness, discomfort, weakness, and treatment-related complications. It is important to listen to your body and modify your exercise levels appropriately, pacing yourself and taking pauses when necessary. Consulting with a healthcare provider may assist in identifying any restrictions or considerations to take while developing an exercise plan.

Finding encouragement from friends, family, or support groups may also help you overcome hurdles to exercise. Having a workout companion or engaging in group activities may help with motivation, accountability, and camaraderie, making exercise more fun and sustainable.

Working With A Healthcare Team To Ensure Safe Exercise

To guarantee safe and successful exercise participation, leukemia patients should consult with a healthcare team including oncologists, nurses, physical therapists, and exercise physiologists. Healthcare practitioners may give personalized advice based on an individual's medical history, treatment regimen, and physical limits.

They may assist in developing a personalized workout program that addresses particular requirements and objectives while minimizing dangers. Regular contact with healthcare experts enables continual monitoring and modifications as required, ensuring that exercise remains a positive and essential component of leukemia treatment.

CHAPTER SEVEN

Stress-Management Techniques

Mindfulness Meditation

Mindfulness meditation is an effective practice for stress reduction and general well-being. It entails concentrating your attention on the current moment without passing judgment, helping you to develop a sense of awareness and acceptance of your thoughts, emotions, and physical sensations.

To practice mindfulness meditation, locate a peaceful and comfortable place where you will not be interrupted. Sit or lay down in a comfortable posture, shut your eyes, and focus on your breath. Consider the feeling of each inhale and exhale, allowing your breath to ground you in the present now.

As you meditate, you may find your thoughts wandering. This is normal. When you realize your mind has wandered, softly return your concentration to your breath without criticizing yourself. With consistent practice, you'll gain increased awareness and the capacity to be present in the face of life's problems.

Deep Breathing Exercises

Deep breathing exercises are another great method for reducing stress and increasing calm. By deliberately slowing your breathing and taking deep, calm breaths, you may trigger your body's natural relaxation reaction.

The 4-7-8 method is a basic deep breathing practice. Begin by sitting comfortably and putting one hand on your belly, and the other on your chest. Inhale deeply through your nose for four counts, and feel your abdomen rise.

Hold your breath for seven counts, then gently exhale through your lips for eight counts, allowing your abdomen to collapse. Repeat this cycle numerous times, concentrating on the rhythm of your breathing.

Deep breathing exercises may be performed whenever and whenever you are worried or overwhelmed. They serve to calm the nervous system, relieve muscular tension, and induce feelings of inner peace and relaxation.

Yoga And Tai Chi For Relaxation

Yoga and Tai Chi are ancient disciplines that use gentle movements, breathwork, and mindfulness to promote relaxation and stress reduction. Both activities have been demonstrated to decrease cortisol levels, lower blood pressure, and boost general happiness and well-being.

Yoga consists of a set of positions, or asanas, done in a fluid sequence, as well as synchronized breathing methods. Tai Chi, on the other hand, is made up of slow, purposeful motions that flow smoothly from one to the next, encouraging balance, flexibility, and inner harmony.

To add yoga or Tai Chi into your stress-management regimen, try taking a class led by a trained teacher or following along with online videos or instructions. Begin with mild, beginner-friendly exercises and progressively raise the intensity as you gain comfort.

Stress Relief Through Creative Activities

Creative hobbies may be a fun and efficient method to reduce stress while also expressing yourself. Painting, sketching, writing, gardening, or playing music are all examples of creative activities that may help you cope with stress and channel your emotions positively.

You do not have to be a professional artist or musician to gain from creative expression. The idea is to just participate in things that make you happy and enable you to express yourself freely and without judgment.

Consider scheduling time each day to pursue a creative hobby or pastime that you like. Experiment with various materials and approaches until you discover what works for you. Remember that the process of producing is just as essential as the outcome, so enjoy the trip rather than strive for perfection.

Seeking Support From Loved Ones

Finally, do not overlook the importance of getting help from loved ones during times of stress. Sharing your thoughts and emotions with trustworthy friends or family members may provide you comfort, perspective, and affirmation, making you feel less alone in your challenges.

Reach out to someone you trust and tell them what you're going through. Whether it's a listening ear, a shoulder to cry on, or practical guidance, having a support system in place may make a huge difference in how you deal with stress and hardship.

Remember that it is OK to seek assistance when necessary and that you do not have to face adversity alone. Surround yourself with people who encourage and support you, and don't be afraid to ask for help when you need it.

CHAPTER EIGHT

The Importance Of Quality Sleep

Understanding Sleep Patterns

Quality sleep is critical to general health and well-being, and understanding sleep patterns is the first step towards obtaining it. Our sleep is separated into three stages: light sleep, deep sleep, and REM sleep. Each step is critical to our physical and mental recovery. Light sleep promotes relaxation, deep sleep is critical for physical repair and development, and REM sleep is necessary for cognitive function and emotional stability.

Keeping a sleep journal might help you better understand your sleep habits. Take note of the time you go to bed, how long it takes you to fall asleep, any interruptions throughout the night, and the time you wake up. Over time, patterns will form that indicate when you are in the various phases of sleep.

This information may help you make changes to enhance the quality of your sleep.

Creating A Restful Sleep Environment

Creating a calm sleep environment is essential for encouraging great sleep. Begin by optimizing your bedroom. Keep it dark, quiet, and cool for better sleep. Invest in a comfy mattress and pillows that can support your body and relieve any pain. Consider using blackout curtains or an eye mask to filter out any exterior light that may interfere with your sleep.

Limit your use of electronic devices before bedtime, since the blue light generated by displays may disrupt your body's normal sleep/wake cycle. Instead, relax by reading or listening to quiet music. Create a nightly ritual to indicate to your body that it is time to relax and prepare for sleep. This might involve taking a warm bath or using relaxation methods like deep breathing or meditation.

Sleep Hygiene Practices

Good sleep hygiene is required for excellent sleep. This includes developing habits and behaviors that encourage good sleep patterns. Consistency is essential, so attempt to go to bed and get up at the same time every day, including weekends. This helps to adjust your body's internal schedule, resulting in greater sleep quality.

Avoid coffee and alcohol close to bedtime since they may interfere with your ability to fall and remain asleep. Similarly, avoid big meals or spicy foods late in the evening, since digestion might interfere with sleep. Create a relaxing nighttime ritual to communicate to your body that it is time to unwind and prepare for sleep.

This might involve reading, taking a warm bath, or practicing relaxation methods like deep breathing or meditation.

Managing Sleep Disturbances

Despite our best efforts, sleep interruptions may still happen. These might include difficulties falling asleep, waking up repeatedly during the night, or waking up too early in the morning. When dealing with sleep difficulties, it is critical to address the root reasons.

Stress and worry are typical causes of sleep problems, therefore developing appropriate stress management strategies is critical. This might involve using relaxation methods like deep breathing or meditation, participating in regular physical exercise, or getting help from a therapist or counselor. Avoiding stimulating activities before bedtime and developing a peaceful evening ritual may also assist in preventing sleep difficulties.

If sleep issues continue, it may be beneficial to visit a medical expert. They can help you discover any underlying medical illnesses or sleep disorders that may be causing your sleep difficulties and offer the best treatment choices.

Seeking Professional Help With Sleep Issues

If you continue to have trouble sleeping after adopting lifestyle modifications, you should seek expert treatment. A sleep medicine specialist may assess your sleep patterns and symptoms to determine if an underlying sleep issue is causing your problems.

Depending on your specific requirements, treatment options may include cognitive-behavioral therapy for insomnia (CBT-I), which addresses negative thinking patterns and behaviors that lead to sleep issues. In rare circumstances, medication may be recommended to assist in normalizing sleep patterns, although this is usually regarded as a temporary remedy.

It is important to discuss freely and honestly with your healthcare physician about your sleep patterns, symptoms, and any concerns you may have. Together, you may create a personalized treatment plan to enhance your sleep quality and general well-being. Remember that getting enough sleep is critical for overall health, and seeking expert assistance is a proactive start towards obtaining it.

CHAPTER NINE

Avoiding Harmful Substances

Effects Of Smoking And Alcohol

Smoking and excessive alcohol use are two behaviors that may have a substantial influence on people's health, particularly those with leukemia. Smoking delivers hazardous substances into the body, raising the risk of several cancers, including leukemia. Furthermore, smoking affects the immune system, making it more difficult for the body to fight infections, which may be especially problematic for leukemia patients with already impaired immune systems.

While alcohol is often used socially, it may also be harmful to leukemia sufferers. Excessive alcohol use might impair the bone marrow's capacity to create blood cells, increasing the symptoms of leukemia and possibly leading to consequences including anemia and an increased susceptibility to infection. Furthermore, drinking might reduce the efficacy of some leukemia drugs, compromising treatment results.

Quitting smoking and reducing alcohol use are critical measures in treating leukemia and increasing general health. Quitting smoking might be difficult, but there are many services and support systems available to assist people break the habit, such as nicotine replacement medicines, counseling, and support groups. Similarly, restricting alcohol use to modest levels, as advised by healthcare specialists, may help reduce its detrimental effects on leukemia and general health.

Risks Of Environmental Toxins

Leukemia sufferers, like everyone else, are constantly exposed to a variety of environmental contaminants. Air pollution, home chemicals, pesticides, and industrial pollutants are all potential sources of these poisons. While it is hard to eradicate environmental contaminants, limiting exposure may help lower the risk of problems for leukemia patients.

Air pollution, for example, includes hazardous particulate matter and chemicals that may aggravate respiratory disorders and impair the immune system, leaving leukemia patients more vulnerable to infections and other health problems. Similarly, home chemicals like cleaning agents and pesticides include dangerous components that may cause damage when breathed or absorbed via the skin.

To decrease their exposure to environmental contaminants, leukemia patients may take many proactive measures. Effective solutions include using natural cleaning products and pesticides, ventilation in interior rooms to enhance air quality, and avoiding high-pollution locations. Wearing protective equipment such as masks and gloves while handling potentially dangerous chemicals may also reduce risk.

Importance Of Medication Compliance

Medication adherence is critical for leukemia patients to properly control their disease and get the best potential results. Leukemia treatment often consists of chemotherapy, targeted therapy, immunotherapy, and supportive drugs, all of which must be given exactly as recommended by healthcare specialists.

Skipping doses or failing to follow medication regimens may reduce treatment effectiveness and raise the risk of illness progression and consequences. Furthermore, many leukemia treatments need regular blood levels to be effective, making compliance even more important.

To ensure drug compliance, leukemia patients should collaborate with their healthcare team to create a thorough treatment plan that includes specific instructions for medication dose, timing, and possible adverse effects. Using pill organizers, setting reminders, and integrating medication regimens into everyday habits may all assist in improving adherence.

Herbal Supplements To Avoid

While herbal supplements are often offered as natural treatments for a variety of health problems, leukemia patients should take care while contemplating their usage. Some herbal supplements may interfere with leukemia treatments or worsen symptoms, jeopardizing treatment efficacy and safety.

Certain herbs, such as echinacea, ginseng, and St. John's wort, may disrupt the metabolism of chemotherapy medications, lowering their effectiveness or raising their toxicity. Furthermore, certain herbal supplements may boost the immune system, which may be dangerous for leukemia patients whose immune systems are already hyperactive.

Before using any herbal supplements, leukemia patients should check with their doctor to verify they are compatible with their treatment regimen. Healthcare providers may offer personalized advice based on an individual's health requirements and possible interactions with leukemia drugs.

Creating A Healthy Environment At Home

Creating a healthy atmosphere at home is critical for promoting leukemia patients' well-being and reducing possible hazards. This includes a variety of tasks, such as maintaining clean indoor air quality, creating a safe and pleasant living environment, and encouraging healthy lifestyle practices for the whole family.

Leukemia patients may enhance indoor air quality by utilizing air purifiers, reducing indoor pollutants like smoking and cooking, and ensuring sufficient ventilation throughout the house. Removing allergens and irritants like dust mites and mold may also assist with respiratory problems and general comfort.

In addition to physical considerations, maintaining a healthy home environment includes promoting emotional and psychological well-being. This might involve establishing areas for relaxation and stress reduction, encouraging open communication within the family, and offering emotional support to help patients deal with the difficulties of leukemia treatment.

Prioritizing a healthy environment at home allows leukemia patients to build a supportive and loving environment that improves their overall quality of life and compliments their medical treatment and lifestyle choices.

CHAPTER TEN

Ensuring Long-Term Health And Wellness

Regular Monitoring And Follow-Up

Regular monitoring and follow-up are critical components of controlling leukemia and ensuring overall health and well-being. Once diagnosed with leukemia, it is critical to create a regimen for monitoring your status and communicating with healthcare experts. This includes frequent check-ups, blood tests, and imaging scans to monitor illness progression and therapy efficacy.

Your healthcare team will work together with you to create a monitoring program that is suited to your individual needs. This might entail regular trips to the doctor's office or the hospital for blood tests and physical exams.

During these sessions, your healthcare practitioner will examine your general health, check your blood cell counts, and look into any symptoms or side effects you are experiencing.

In addition to medical monitoring, you should pay attention to your body and report any changes or concerns to your healthcare provider right away. This proactive strategy may help detect possible difficulties early on and prevent complications from escalating.

Regular monitoring and follow-up also allow you to address any changes to your treatment plan or lifestyle suggestions. You may improve your leukemia management and long-term health and well-being by remaining connected with your healthcare team and actively engaging in your treatment.

Changing Diet And Lifestyle Over Time

Leukemia management requires a comprehensive strategy that involves both medical therapy and lifestyle changes such as diet and exercise. As you go through your leukemia treatment, it's important to remember that your dietary and lifestyle demands may vary over time, and modifications may be required to maintain your overall health and wellness.

One of the most important factors when changing your diet is ensuring that you get enough nourishment to support your immune system and energy levels. Depending on your treatment plan and personal health, you may need to adjust your food intake to ensure you obtain enough calories, protein, vitamins, and minerals. This may include consulting with a licensed dietitian, who may give tailored dietary advice based on your unique requirements and preferences.

In addition to diet, you should prioritize physical activity and exercise as part of your daily routine. Regular exercise may help you improve your strength, endurance, and general quality of life, even when you are undergoing leukemia treatment. However, before beginning any new fitness program, you should contact your healthcare provider to verify it is safe and suitable for your specific needs.

It's typical to notice changes in your nutritional choices, energy levels, and physical capacities as you deal with the ups and downs of leukemia treatment. By being adaptable, you may gradually alter your food and lifestyle to meet these changes while still supporting your long-term health and wellness.

Finding Joy In Everyday Life

Living with leukemia may be difficult, but it is essential to find moments of pleasure and enjoyment in daily situations.

Finding pleasure does not imply dismissing the facts of your condition or downplaying the challenges you may encounter. Instead, it's about living in the present now, practicing appreciation, and seeking out activities and experiences that offer you joy and fulfillment.

One method to find pleasure in daily life is to concentrate on what you can manage while appreciating the tiny moments of beauty and connection that surround you. This might be spending quality time with loved ones, engaging in hobbies or interests, or just taking time to relax and rejuvenate.

Mindfulness and gratitude practices may also help you develop a feeling of pleasure and fulfillment in your everyday life. By deliberately concentrating on the present moment and expressing thankfulness for what you have, you may change your perspective and discover purpose and fulfillment even amid hardship.

It's also important to allow oneself to feel a variety of emotions, such as grief, rage, and frustration, without judgment. Accepting and accepting your emotions helps you to process them healthily and creates room for pleasure and happiness to arise.

Finally, finding pleasure in daily life is a personal journey that takes various forms for each individual. By identifying what makes you happy and making time for it, you may create a feeling of pleasure and well-being that will get you through the difficulties of living with leukemia.

Celebrating Progress And Achievements

Living with leukemia entails negotiating several hurdles and milestones along the road. It is important to celebrate your progress and accomplishments, no matter how modest, as you strive to preserve your health and well-being.

Every step forward, whether it is finishing a cycle of treatment, achieving a personal goal, or just getting through a tough day, needs to be recognized and celebrated. Acknowledging your successes may enhance your confidence, enthusiasm, and feeling of empowerment while you continue your leukemia treatment.

Setting and tracking reasonable objectives that reflect your beliefs and priorities is one approach to celebrating achievement. These objectives might be health-related, such as sticking to a regular workout regimen or reaching a certain nutritional milestone, or they can be personal, bringing you pleasure and fulfillment.

It's also important to acknowledge the help and encouragement you've received from loved ones, carers, and healthcare experts along the road. Their wisdom, sympathy, and steadfast support are invaluable in your leukemia journey and deserve to be recognized and thanked.

Celebrating progress and successes entails not just appreciating how far you've gone, but also being encouraged and inspired to keep going ahead. By reflecting on your accomplishments and expressing thanks to those who support you, you may create a feeling of resilience and positivity that will carry you through the ups and downs of living with leukemia.

Continuing Education And Support Network

Living with leukemia requires continuous learning and adjustment to new knowledge, therapies, and problems. Continuing education enables you to make educated choices about your health and well-being while also advocating for yourself successfully.

Your healthcare team, which includes physicians, nurses, and other medical experts who care for you, is an excellent source of continuing education. Do not be afraid to ask questions, seek clarification, and be educated about your diagnosis, treatment choices, and any possible side effects or problems.

In addition to healthcare experts, support networks may provide vital knowledge, assistance, and encouragement as you navigate your leukemia journey. This might include support groups, online forums, or peer mentorship programs where you can interact with individuals who understand your situation and exchange experiences and ideas.

Continuing education also includes maintaining current on the latest research and innovations in leukemia therapy and management. This may include reading credible materials, attending educational events or conferences, and being involved with advocacy groups committed to leukemia research and awareness.

By actively seeking knowledge and assistance, you may empower yourself to make better health choices, handle problems more successfully, and advocate for the treatment and resources you need to flourish. Continuing education is a constant process that unfolds as you learn and progress during your entire journey.

CONCLUSION

To summarise, the influence of food and lifestyle choices on leukemia, although not a direct cause, is increasingly seen as important in controlling the illness and enhancing general health. While no one diet will cure leukemia, eating a balanced, nutrient-dense diet may help the body fight the illness and deal with treatment side effects.

A diet high in fruits, vegetables, whole grains, lean meats, and healthy fats may supply the vital nutrients and antioxidants required to sustain immune function, reduce inflammation, and promote general health. Additionally, keeping hydrated and avoiding excessive intake of processed meals, sugary snacks, and alcohol may help to improve well-being.

Furthermore, lifestyle choices such as regular physical exercise, stress management strategies, and appropriate sleep are critical in helping leukemia patients maintain immunological function, reduce tiredness, and improve their overall quality of life.

While more study is required to completely understand the complicated relationship between nutrition, lifestyle, and leukemia, adopting healthy behaviors may supplement medical therapy by empowering patients to better control their illness and optimize their health results. Taking a comprehensive strategy that considers both medical and lifestyle aspects is critical for enhancing the well-being and quality of life of leukemia patients.

THE END

www.ingramcontent.com/pod-product-compliance
Lightning Source LLC
Chambersburg PA
CBHW071836210526
45479CB00001B/160